A Beginner's Guide to Pickleball

Moon Webster

Table of Contents

Introduction

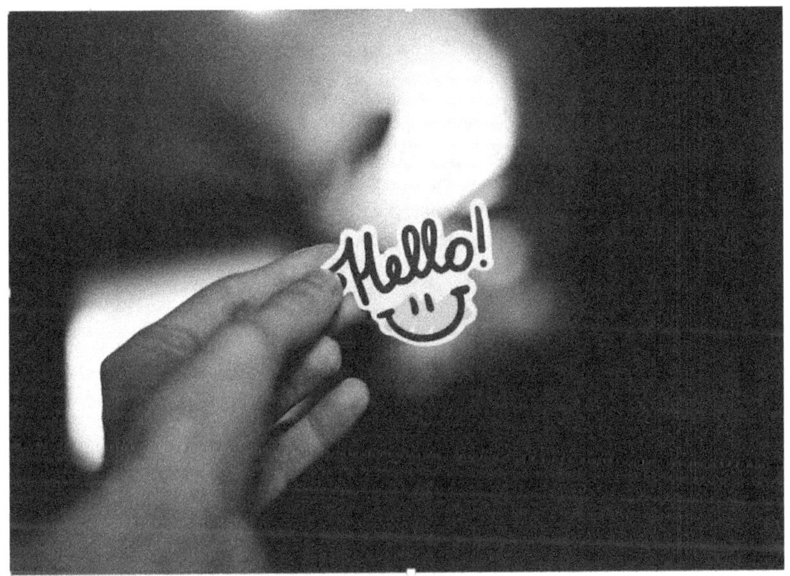

The conception of pickleball can be traced back to 1965 when it was created on an island in proximity to Seattle, Washington. Due to their usual summer activities becoming monotonous, the three fathers, namely Joel Pritchard, Bill Bell, and Barney McCallum, came together and established the concept for the game. If your desire is to understand the beginnings of pickleball on a tiny island in Washington over 50 years ago, then watching the video would be advisable.

Pickleball's popularity is rapidly growing, with an increasing number of countries participating in the sport. People of diverse age ranges and fitness abilities derive enjoyment from engaging in racket sports. Similarly to Ping-Pong, pickleball utilizes a paddle; however, it incorporates elements from both tennis and badminton.

Over the years, it has gained significant popularity as a sport in both the United States and Canada. Countries on other continents, such as Europe and Asia, are also adopting the game's popularity and are constructing additional courts (*Introduction to Pickleball, 2023*).

Tournaments and organizations have started proliferating, with an increasing number of individuals expressing interest. Amid the 2020 lockdown, individuals sought fresh methods of keeping fit and engaged, leading to a surge in the popularity of pickleball. Originally just a recreational activity played in people's backyards, this sport has now gained enough momentum that it is being considered for inclusion in the Olympic Games within a few years.

What factors contribute to the widespread appeal of pickleball? One reason for its appeal is that it allows for play in both indoor and outdoor settings, and it accommodates either two or four players. Additionally, mastering the rules of the game is a straightforward process for newcomers, who can quickly grasp its mechanics. As your skills improve and you gain knowledge of new tactics, the game can also be played in a competitive manner and at a quicker tempo. Additionally, as in the past, pickleball is played using simple equipment.

In addition to being highly enjoyable, pickleball distinguishes itself from sports like tennis by its quick learning curve and the potential for rapid skill improvement without the need for formal lessons. You can play pickleball at your nearby park or even in your backyard if it's large enough. Normally, it is played on a court the size of a badminton court, but some people have been managing with smaller spaces (Nelson, 2021).

In the course of its development, pickleball has also undergone transformations and advancements, including the creation of specialized gear such as paddles and footwear designed exclusively for the sport. You also don't have to wear expensive sports clothes. All you need to play is a sturdy paddle, usually made of wood, a perforated ball made of a special material, and a net that is not very high.

Another reason why pickleball has become so popular in more recent years is because it is a social sport. In Pickleball, there is the option to play with a team or with only two participants (Macpherson, 2023). With gyms and fitness centers having been closed for almost a whole year, people also had to find new ways to stay active. In ensuing years, many of us have become bored of doing online workout classes and want to try something else. Also, because pickleball is not a sport where people touch each other, you can still play and follow the social distancing rules to which we've become accustomed.

For both adults and children, pickleball has become the fastest-growing sport in the United States. The game has gained recognition as a social sport mainly because it cultivates team dynamics and provides a great deal of fun. With its wide acclaim, it's even gaining momentum among elderly individuals in retirement communities.

My intention with this guide is to elaborate on the fundamental aspects of this incredible sport and emphasize its exceptional features. And who knows, it may be something that you will think about starting yourself or introducing to your children!

Chapter 1: Welcome to the Wonderful World of Pickleball!

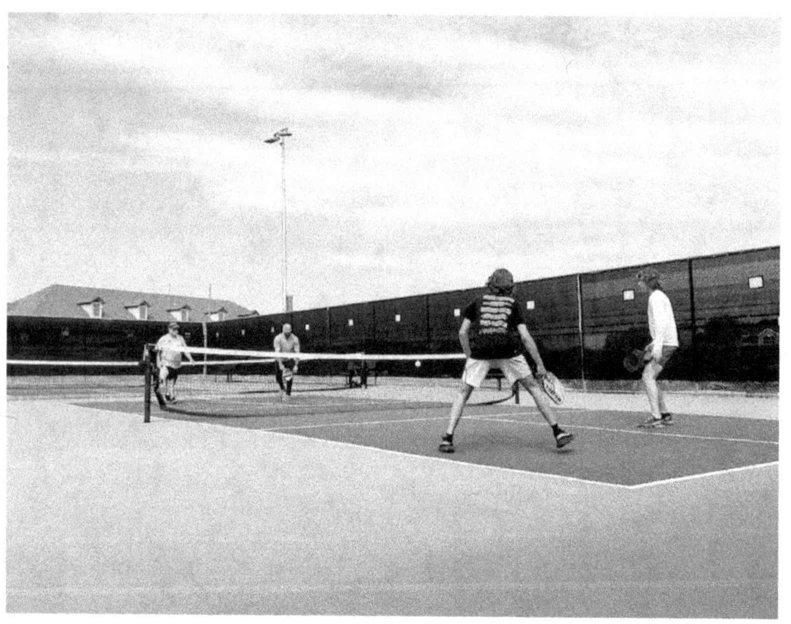

The focus of this chapter will be on an exhilarating sport that is gaining popularity among individuals worldwide. If you are new to pickleball or want to enhance your abilities, I am here to guide you in learning and comprehending the game.

Pickleball's rise in popularity can be attributed, in part, to its straightforward nature. People who are beginners and want to start off with something uncomplicated will find this a fantastic choice as its rules are straightforward and easy to grasp. By combining elements from tennis, badminton, and Ping-Pong, pickleball offers a distinctive play experience and involves the use of a paddle and a plastic ball with perforations.

Regardless of your age or level of expertise, this sport provides a fun and effortless activity for everyone to partake in. With the option to play either indoors or outdoors, the game further caters to a wide range of people by allowing anyone, anywhere to participate. The limited equipment needed will also help you save money, as pickleball is a game that involves only a paddle and a ball.

The size of the court is smaller than a tennis court, with dimensions of 20 ft by 44 ft, and a net divides it into two separate sections. To begin a game, a player hits the ball at an angle to the opposition player. Before players can begin hitting the ball back and forth, it is necessary for them to ensure that it bounces once on their side and then on the opposing side.

The objective is to successfully strike the ball across the net and within the limits of the court, avoiding hitting it outside of bounds or into the net. Point scoring occurs when the opponent fails to make a good return of the ball. You can engage in a game of pickleball either with one person per team or with two individuals per team. In singles matches, one player competes against another player, whereas in doubles matches, two players compete together against another team.

The sport is both exhilarating and gratifying. Indulging in this action sparks your drive to achieve victory while also providing an enjoyable and positive experience. Furthermore, being physically active serves as a great benefit to your overall well-being. Engaging in pickleball, while centered around competition, provides people with a lighthearted opportunity to bond with one another. The game's pleasant design facilitates effortless communication and friendship-building among fellow players.

While the strategies and operational mechanisms may vary across different formats, the fundamental principles of the game remain unchanged. Having the appropriate technique and footwork is of utmost importance, similar to any other sport. Improving your performance can be achieved through consistent practice and honing your swing technique and court movement. By regularly practicing techniques and engaging in friendly matches, you will witness improvement in your performance and develop a greater sense of confidence while playing.

Whether you're engaged in recreational playing or involved in a competitive event, you will always experience fellowship and sincerity. Combining physical prowess with strategic thinking, pickleball offers a delightful and inclusive sporting experience.

As you begin your pickleball journey, make sure to find joy in the game, keep yourself active, and appreciate its growing popularity.

Chapter 2: Getting Started With Pickleball

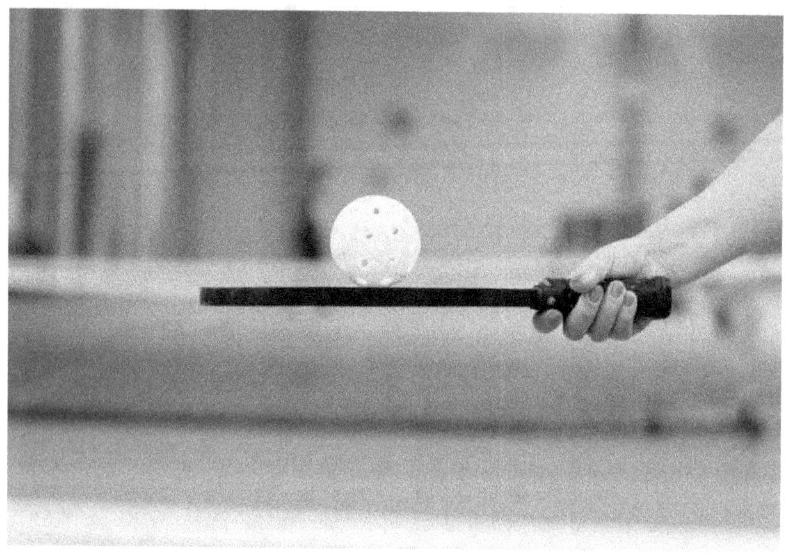

Before you start playing pickleball, it is essential to gather the necessary equipment.

In order to play, it is essential to have a paddle. Typically constructed from materials such as graphite, fiberglass, or wood, these paddles are smaller in size compared to tennis rackets and they feature a solid surface. To ensure optimal maneuverability and control, it is important for the paddle's handle to feel comfortable and easy to move.

After that, you will need the pickleballs. Available in various colors, these balls are specifically designed for the sport. A regular Wiffle ball is heavier and has larger openings compared to these, which are lighter and have smaller openings.

Pickleball sets are also available for purchase at any retailer specializing in sports gear. The set is composed of paddles and balls, making it ideal for beginners in the sport.

Now that you're prepared with the right equipment, it's time to locate a court where you can play pickleball. The dimensions of pickleball courts are smaller compared to tennis courts and have their own specific measurements. Similar to a tennis court, the pickleball court is divided into two sections by a net. The entire area of each section is divided into two segments—one where you must wait for the ball to bounce before hitting it, and another where you have the freedom to play without any restrictions.

Stretching 7 ft on each side, the former area referred to as the "kitchen" or "non-volley zone" is present on either side. While the ball is airborne, it is prohibited to strike it in this designated region, which features on either side of the net.

The game commences once someone initiates the serve with the ball. The goal is to hit the ball over the net and into the other person's side to try to get points. One side tries to hit the ball back while the opposing team strives to prevent them from doing so.

To initiate the game, take a stance at the back boundary of the court and lightly tap the ball with your hand, ensuring it stays below your waist. Make certain the ball is successfully propelled across the net and accurately lands in the corner of the court situated at the opposite end. The serve must be executed with a diagonal motion, similar to tennis. Once the game has commenced, players are allowed to strike the ball either upward or after it has touched the ground. However, it is important to bear in mind that hitting the ball within the non-volley zone is only allowed after it has bounced.

In the early stages of playing pickleball, it is vital to dedicate your efforts to becoming proficient at the game and grasping its strategic elements. To improve your ability to manipulate the ball, ensure to engage in diverse drills that involve striking the ball. This means striking it using your forehand, striking it using your backhand, and striking it while it's airborne without allowing it to touch the ground. To maximize your influence during the game, pay attention to your footwork and court positioning.

Ensure to engage in continual practice and seek help from seasoned players. This helpful tip will assist you in enhancing your abilities and improving your proficiency. Practice being kind and patient with yourself while learning the sport, and don't put excessive pressure on yourself if it takes more time to grasp. Everyone learns at their own speed.

Don't forget to have fun and enjoy yourself at all times. Experience the joy of playing alongside others, forging new connections, and embracing pure happiness throughout this delightful game. It is my utmost priority to underscore the sheer enthusiasm I have for ensuring that all of you simply have fun while playing the sport. Once you acknowledge and value that specific aspect, you will become aware of the considerable improvements and progress you have made and will continue to achieve.

Now that you're armed with a good foundation in the essentials of pickleball, it is the perfect time to head to the court and initiate gameplay. So, get your paddle, grab some balls, and let the pickleball fun commence!

Chapter 3: Rules and Regulations

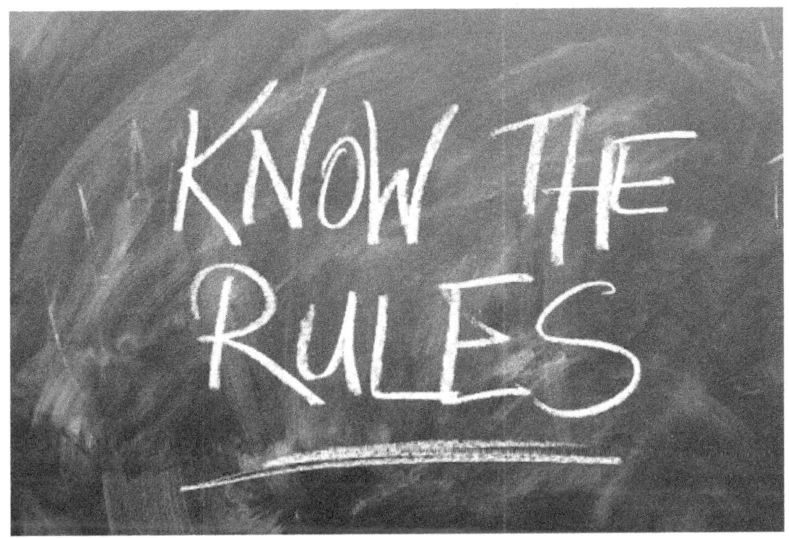

To fully enjoy and grasp the game of pickleball, it's important to become acquainted with the rules and regulations that govern this fun sport. Adhering to these guidelines ensures that all players engage in fair play and enjoy their time on the court.

As mentioned in Chapter 2, the dimensions of a typical pickleball court are slightly smaller when compared to those of a tennis court. The court is divided into two sections by a net, the height of which measures 36 in. at the center and 34 in. on the edges. It is essential to keep in mind that the net must not touch the ground while playing as this could lead to issues arising during the game.

To adhere to the rules, the person serving must maintain the placement of both of their feet behind the line situated at the back of the court. It is forbidden for players to make contact with the ball while it is airborne within the designated non-volley area on the court. When a player violates this rule, it is regarded as a fault.

Remembering the double-bounce rule is of utmost importance. Once the ball bounces for the first time, both teams can decide to either strike the ball before it bounces again or allow another bounce. There are no regulations on how to hit the ball after each team has hit it twice, allowing them to continue hitting it freely.

Points are scored in pickleball when you successfully hit or serve the ball over the net and prevent your opponent from returning it. Points can be scored if your opponent hits the ball outside the designated area. Each player takes turns serving the ball, and scoring points is solely allowed for the team currently serving. The first team or player to achieve the required number of points and maintain a lead of two points emerges as the winner. In the absence of a two-point lead, the game will proceed.

In summary, here is a simple breakdown of the five basic rules of pickleball:

- Hitting the ball outside the confines of the playing area is prohibited.

- To serve the ball, you need to use your hand, kept underneath your waistline, and hit the ball.

- To successfully serve in a game, the ball needs to hit the ground, first on the opposition's side and subsequently on the server's side, before being struck back to the opponent. After the ball has bounced twice, players can hit it in the air.

- When you serve in a game, you need to make sure your ball doesn't land in a specific area called the non-volley zone.

- To emerge as the victor, you must achieve a score of either 11, 15, or 21 points. Typically, players aim to achieve 11 points as their primary goal. A 2-point advantage is required for you to be in the lead (Macpherson, 2023).

Playing pickleball necessitates being a good sport and adhering to the rules. Show respect and be polite to your opponents and referees, and refrain from behaving unjustly or disrespecting others. It is important to keep in mind that pickleball should be an enjoyable and inclusive game. Hence, always play with honesty and fairness.

Once you grasp and comply with these instructions, you will be fully equipped to engage in a fun-filled game of pickleball. Grab your paddle, step onto the court, and encounter the electrifying domain of pickleball.

Chapter 4: Equipment and Apparel

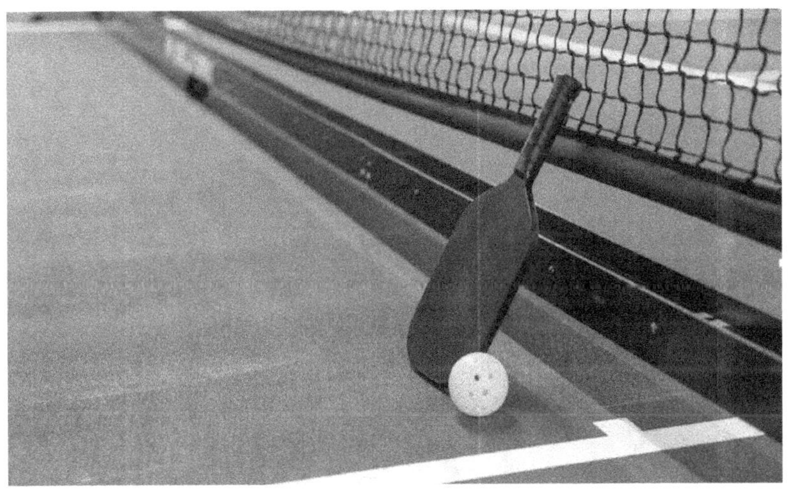

Playing any sport, including pickleball, requires the appropriate equipment and clothing. Numerous items are available for purchase to enhance your performance in the game. These things include the following items.

Shoes

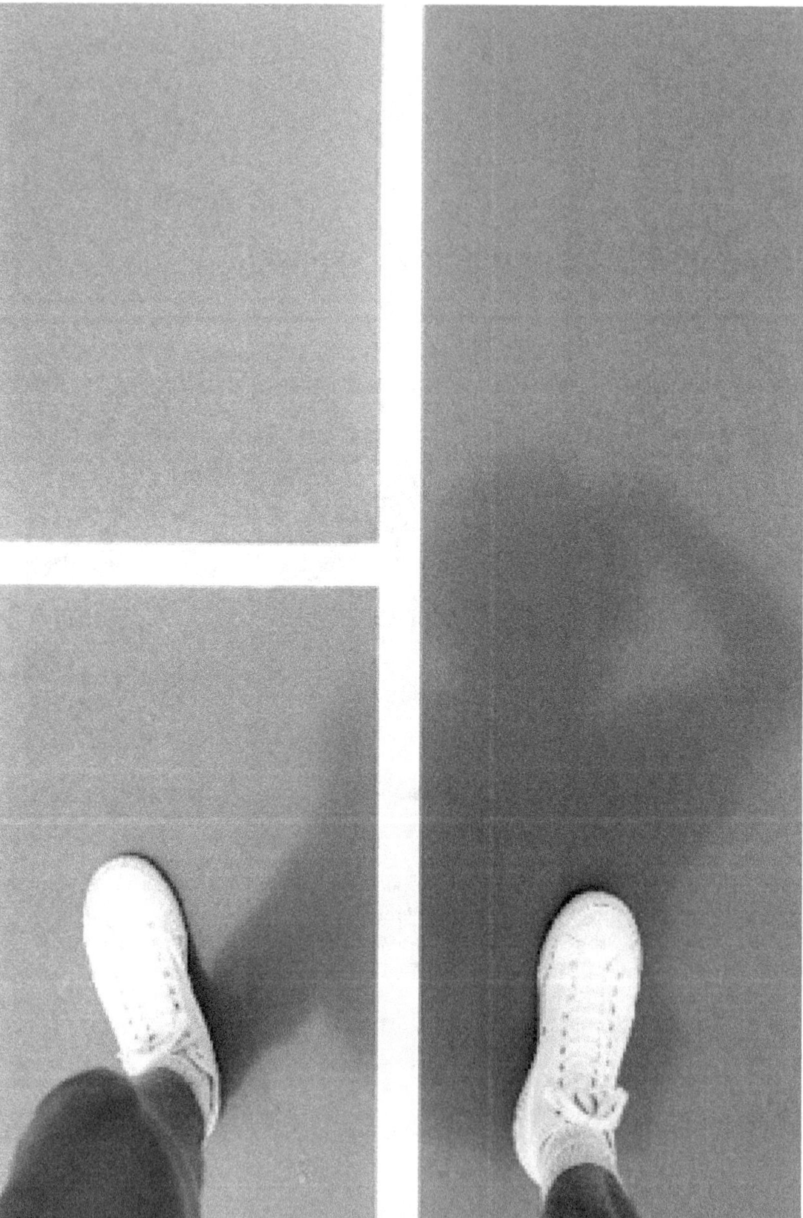

The correct footwear plays a vital role in every sport. Wearing specific footwear for pickleball is not mandatory, but it is recommended to wear shoes that are appropriate for playing on a court. The shoes must offer excellent sideways support while also being lightweight. These requirements are met by the production of specific pickleball shoes. Wearing tennis shoes is also beneficial for this activity. Important features to consider when searching for pickleball shoes include that they:

- are slip-resistant and do not leave marks on surfaces

- have nice support for the curve of your foot

- have mesh that allows air to flow easily

- offer heel stability, meaning they are steady and secure for your heel while you are walking or standing

- possess good traction, meaning that they have a strong grip or connection to the ground or surface they are on

- have a shock absorbing midsole, which is a part of a shoe that helps cushion and protect the feet from impact and sudden shocks

- are the right size for your feet

Paddles

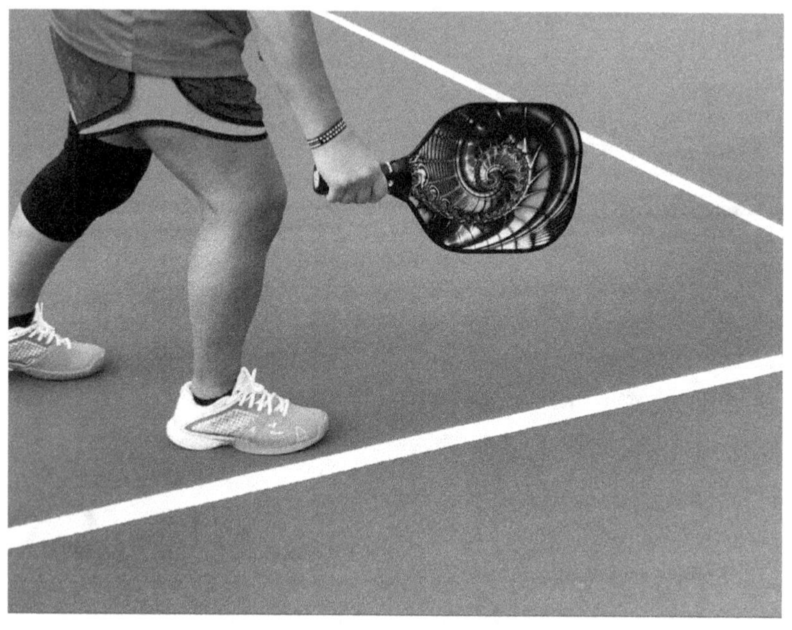

In order to engage in pickleball, you must possess a paddle. There is a plethora of paddle choices available in various sizes and types. The size of the face, surface area, roughness, durability and strength, weight, adequacy of hitting area, controllability, and holding-area comfort are all essential aspects to consider when seeking a paddle.

Paddles can be constructed using a variety of materials including wood, graphite, plastic, carbon fiber, and fiberglass. A carbon fiber option costs more money but is lighter, softer, and lasts longer. It also helps you maintain better control of the ball, but your hit won't be as strong.

Fiberglass paddles are cheaper and can offer you more strength when you use them. If you have a problem with having enough strength, then a paddle made of this material might be the most suitable option.

Graphite paddles are light and strong. They have a solid surface that helps players hit quick shots and respond faster. These paddles also cost less money than other materials.

Pick a paddle that is right for your playing style, considering whether you want more control or more power. You should also think about how big the paddle is and make sure it fits your hand.

Balls

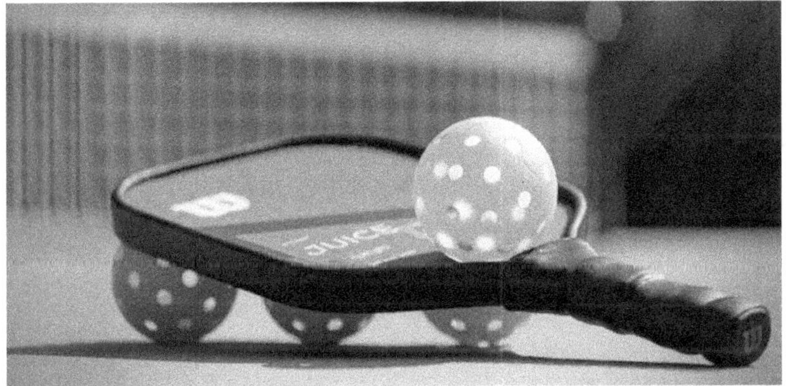

Pickleballs resemble Wiffle balls in appearance as they are constructed with smooth plastic material and feature varying sizes of holes on the exterior. They come in different colors like yellow, black, pink, blue, and more. A good pickleball should have a nice bounce and be neither too easy to hit nor easily breakable. Very solid balls stay usable for the longest time, but they may not hit as effectively as softer ones.

Indoor and outdoor balls are different because they have a different number of holes in them. Indoor balls have 26 big holes each while outdoor balls have 40 small holes each. Balls used outdoors are usually heavier and firmer compared to those used indoors. This is because they need to be able to travel further and withstand the elements for a longer period of time.

Apparel

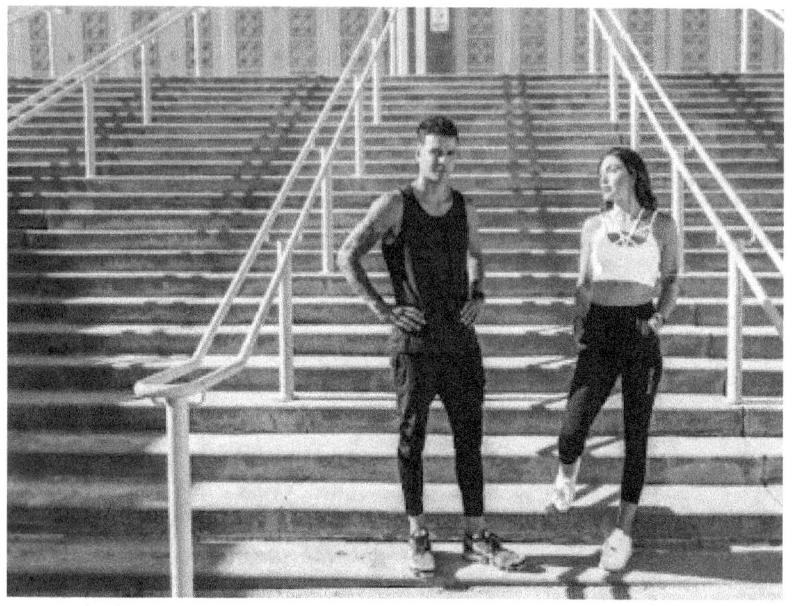

When shopping for sportswear, it's worth considering options that are not overly baggy and that aid in sweat absorption. Look for bags or totes that have shock-absorption capabilities and are designed to accommodate your equipment. Search for accessories that are specifically designed to accommodate your ball bands. Also keep a water bottle with your equipment and seek out hats or visors that have the capacity to absorb sweat while also providing eye protection against the sun. While engaging in pickleball, numerous individuals opt to wear goggles or safety glasses for eye protection (Macpherson, 2023).

While pickleball typically poses minimal risk, accidents can still happen, underscoring the need for being prepared. For preventive purposes, a number of players use wristbands or elbow pads to shield themselves from potential harm. Shock-absorbing sports bras are also a good idea.

Having the appropriate gear and attire is crucial for an enjoyable pickleball experience. Prior to engaging in this sport, it's essential to ensure you have all the necessary equipment. With everything you need, playing this thrilling game can provide you with a genuinely enjoyable experience.

Chapter 5: Basic Strokes and Tactics

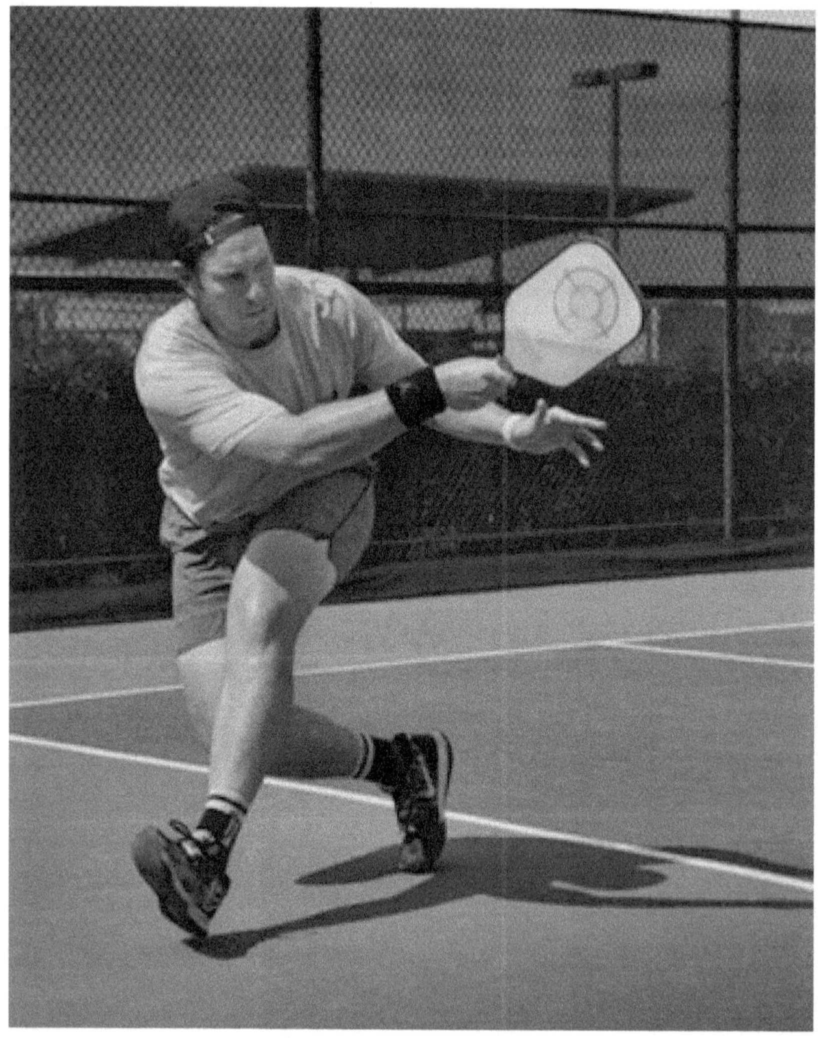

To succeed in a competitive pickleball match, beginners must familiarize themselves with the fundamental techniques of basic shots. The ball can be hit using various strokes, providing different ways of playing the game. Although the number of actions is limited, there are necessary steps that must be followed prior to capturing a shot.

Acquiring proficiency in the shots is something I will discuss that will enable you to thoroughly enjoy your pickleball experience. From this point, you can develop your abilities and keep getting better. I will categorize and explore the different kinds of strokes and shots that you need to familiarize yourself with below.

Typical Strokes to Comply With

Because the stroke happens before the shot, it is logical for me to talk about this first. There are three main types of strokes: groundstrokes, volleys, and dinks.

- **Groundstrokes:** A groundstroke is any shot made after the ball has bounced. This is the simplest type of stroke that you will play, where you hit most of your shots while standing on the ground. However, as in tennis, there are two main ways to hit the ball: using the front of your hand (forehand) or using the back of your hand (backhand).

    - Forehand groundstrokes: People use forehand groundstrokes frequently because they are good for hitting the ball accurately and with power. They will usually be used very near the bottom line of the court.

    - Backhand groundstrokes: Surprisingly, backhand groundstrokes are the strokes that the majority of players use the most. The ideal time to use it is whenever the ball is coming toward your arm and you are not supporting or holding your paddle tightly against it.

- **Volleys:** The act of volleying occurs when the ball is struck without making contact with the ground. The shot's position is irrelevant in this scenario. As long as it hasn't been rejected, then everything is in order. Due to the ball's continued aerial trajectory and increased momentum, these strokes generally exhibit greater strength and power. To play volleys, it is essential to acquire knowledge, practice frequently, and be prepared for these upcoming challenges.

- **Dinks:** This kind of stroke is like a soft whisper because it doesn't have a lot of force. To play a dink, you will strike the ball near the net in the kitchen area of the court. The objective is to hit the ball over the net and distract your opponent, causing them to lose concentration. Successfully executing this shot from a distance in your court can prove challenging, but if done correctly, it has the potential to cause your opponent to falter.

Typical Shots to Comply With

To excel in pickleball, it is essential to acquire proficiency in several renowned techniques of the game. Below are a few of the top moves that are highly favored and recommended for mastery. By putting in the effort to practice and become proficient in these shots, you will have the ability to advance to the more intricate shots commonly employed by professionals and advanced players.

- **Serving the ball:** While the act of serving in pickleball may not be particularly thrilling, it remains a vital aspect of the game and should not be overlooked. Before any other shots can be made, a game must start with a serve, which is the first shot.

- **Drive hits:** The primary aim of executing a drive hit is to generate power and strike the ball with the utmost strength. In a normal game, it is advisable to avoid excessive use of the hit and instead reserve it for offensive moves. When you observe an open area on the other player's side, it can be an advantageous moment to hit the ball with power. The concept is that the hit will come too fast for them to send it back. It is beneficial to have an available entry point because it would require an opponent to rush and attempt to pass through it. Alternatively, it could be beneficial to hit the ball with force and create distance if your opponents are advancing toward you because it becomes more challenging for them to deliver powerful hits when they are busy moving.

- **Lobs:** A lob shot, also referred to as a lofted shot, involves hitting the ball high toward the back of your opponent's court. When done correctly, it makes your opponent attack and move to the back of their playing area, providing you with a chance to unwind and prepare yourself for the next step. If your opponent has to hastily chase a ball, there is a higher chance of them making errors or feeling anxious. This is why players love to use lobs in pickleball. However, be cautious as your speed will be essential if your adversary successfully returns the ball.

- **The block:** In case you're unsure about how to put an end to or regulate the abovementioned shots and movements, I can put it in simpler terms for you—the block shot is the solution you need. This move is not difficult to execute and has the potential to slow down any game. It also has the potential to provide you with an edge once more. To hit the ball:

  - raise your paddle in a backhanded position; you only need to do that and then stop hitting the ball and not move your paddle anymore.

  - next, raise the paddle to the right position and let your movement help you. When done correctly, the ball should go slightly above the net and land in your opponent's kitchen area.

  This shot will be hard for players to hit back because the ball is dropping softly and doesn't have much extra power.

- **Your hit:** These are the different kinds of hits and moves that any new pickleball player should concentrate on when starting the sport. After learning the basic shots, the third drop shot, centerline ace, or the fake dink will be much easier to understand and become skilled at. Remember these moves and shots the next time you play pickleball. If you want to start playing, now is your opportunity to learn the skills talked about in the article "The Strokes and Shots of Pickleball" (2021) and start your pickleball adventure.

Don't forget, getting really good at the basic moves and strategies in pickleball takes time and practice that never stops. To get better at something like playing a game, it's important to practice often and ask experienced players for advice. This will help you become more skilled. If you work hard and keep trying, you will become a really good pickleball player who can handle anything on the court.

Chapter 6: Scoring and Strategy

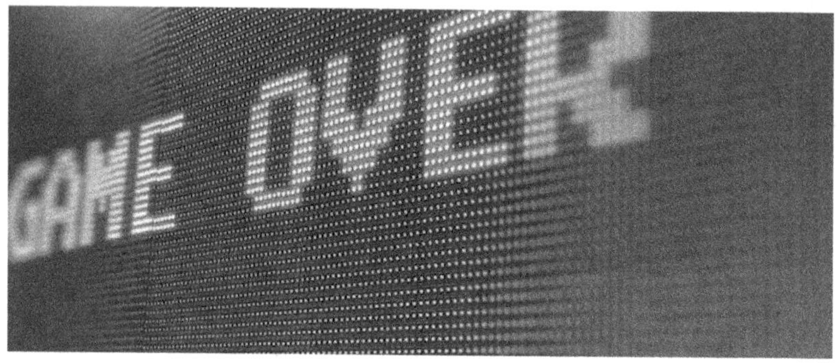

Knowing how points are earned and utilizing sound strategies are essential for performing well in a game. Delving into the workings of scoring and exploring diverse approaches to enhance your gaming abilities will be my primary objective in this chapter.

To begin with, it is important to understand the scoring protocol in pickleball. Like in tennis, you get points when the other team can't hit the ball back into the designated area. The game is initiated by the server who strikes the ball diagonally across the net, aiming to land it within the opposing team's zone.

The rally keeps going until someone makes a mistake or the ball goes outside of the playing area. In order to get a point, the team that is serving needs to win a round. However, only the team that is currently serving can earn points. If the team that receives the ball wins a round, they don't get a point, but they do get to serve the ball next. This special way of scoring makes the game more strategic because keeping the serve becomes essential.

Now, let's learn some important tactics that will help you improve your performance on the pickleball court.

A very important strategy is to focus on being consistent rather than trying to be powerful. Although it might feel good to swing the paddle as hard as possible, concentrating on control and accuracy will earn you better outcomes. The goal is to hit the ball in places that are hard for your opponents to hit back instead of just using strong shots.

Another thing to understand in strategy is how important the dink shot is. The dink shot is performed when you hit the ball gently over the net and near the other team's baseline. This shot helps you force your opponents to make mistakes or hit weak shots. Learning how to do a dink shot really well can give you a big advantage when you play in competitive matches.

In the game of pickleball, communicating and collaborating as a team is essential. Having a strong comprehension of court movement, shot selection, and positioning is crucial for effective communication and synergy with your partner. To manage this, develop a means of co-ordinating actions and employing and during gameplay by utilizing signals or verbal communication. Enhancing communication skills fosters a deeper understanding between you and your partner, ultimately resulting in improved teamwork and increased success.

Ultimately, the capability to adjust and alter is of utmost significance in pickleball. Study your opponents' strengths and weaknesses and change your plan accordingly. If you see that your opponents are having trouble with hitting low shots, try to use more drop shots during the game. If they don't like fast rallies, make your shots faster and stronger. Being able to change and adjust easily will surprise your opponents and give you an advantage.

To sum up, if you want to do really well at pickleball, it's important to know how the scoring system works and come up with effective strategies to use. If you want to win on the court, try to be consistent, practice the dink shot, work on communication and teamwork, and be flexible. Grab your paddle, venture onto the court, and utilize scoring and strategy to ensure your success in pickleball.

Chapter 7: Serving and Receiving

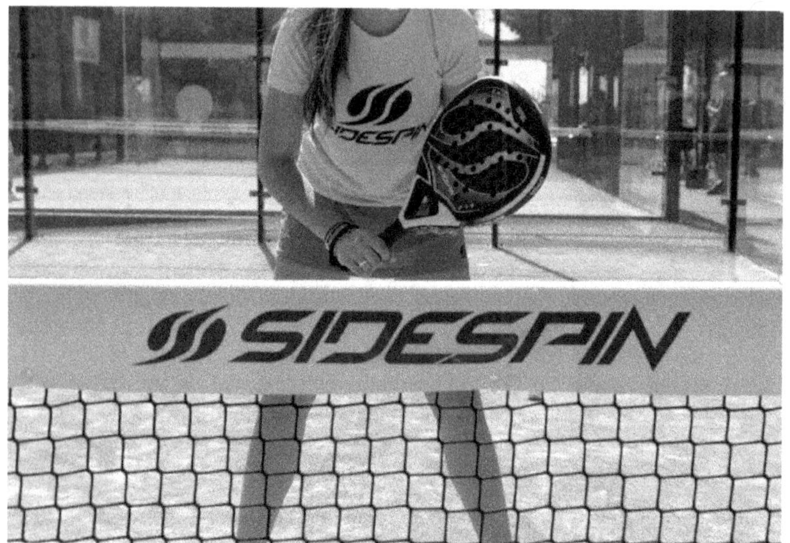

In order to perform well, I must emphasize that it is crucial to have a comprehensive understanding of the rules and techniques associated with pickleball. These have been listed in the previous chapters. In this chapter on this fast-paced sport, my focus will be on the crucial aspects of serving and receiving. Achieving success in competitive pickleball and finding pure enjoyment in the game requires that players master both of these essential skills.

Serving

Let's begin with serving.

The server initiates every rally, and this establishes the atmosphere for the entire point. Opponents tend to be pushed into a defensive position when faced with a powerful serve. The serve needs to be executed by hand, and the paddle should be held lower than your waist. To execute the serve in the game, you need to position yourself at the back of the court and hit the ball at an angle toward the other side, ensuring it lands within the appropriate region of the opponent's court.

The person serving the ball must not hit the net and must hit the ball past a certain area before the other team can hit it back. It is important to study the correct methods to make your serving game better. One important element is to find the correct way to hold your paddle. There are three standard grips in pickleball:

- **Continental grip:** The continental grip, also known as the hammer grip, is the grip that professional players use most often. Its appeal lies in its ability to make hitting different types of shots relatively effortless.

- **Eastern grip:** The eastern grip is a popular and easy way to grip the paddle. You can make it even more stable by extending one of your fingers. This grip is easy for beginners and helps you learn how to use the continental grip.

- **Western grip:** The western grip is another way to hold the paddle that makes it easier to hit forehand shots.

To find the best way to hold your paddle and play comfortably, you will need to try different methods and see what feels right for you.

How to Find a Grip That Works for You

- **Eastern grip**: Hold the paddle in front of you with one hand while using your other hand to hold the flat part of the paddle. This way, you can see the thin side of the paddle. Put the hand that holds your paddle on the front side. Move your hand down the flat part until you're holding the handle like you would hold someone's hand.

- **Continental grip**: Hold the paddle using the eastern grip and turn your wrist either a bit to the left if you are right-handed or a bit to the right if you are left-handed. Position your thumb and index finger in a v-shape, directing them toward the side that is opposite your paddle.

- **Western grip**: To hold the paddle with the western grip, if you happen to be right-handed, simply twist your wrist 90° to the right. Conversely, if you are left-handed, twist it 90° in the direction of the left (Macpherson, 2023).

I recommend the continental grip. There is a reason this is the most popular way for players to hold the paddle when they serve in pickleball: It gives you more power and flexibility in where you aim your shot. However, try using different ways of holding the paddle to see which one feels the best and most like how you would normally hold something.

The Toss

Another important factor when serving is the toss. To toss the ball properly, you need to be able to do it the same way every time. This will help you aim well and hit the ball accurately. Keep throwing the ball to the same place every time you serve, making sure it is the right height and distance from where you want to hit it.

When you hit the ball, try to use a gentle and co-ordinated movement. Keep your paddle slightly open and hit the ball when it's at its highest point. This will make the ball spin a lot when you serve and will help you maintain more control over it. Make sure to aim well and hit your target every time you serve.

Receiving

Now that I have talked about serving, let's move on to receiving.

The team that receives the serve wants to send the ball back in order to have the advantage in the game. Having good receiving skills can help you get ahead and derail your opponent's strategy.

When you receive the ball, it is crucial to stay attentive and be prepared to respond rapidly. Place yourself in the middle of the baseline so that you have a fair chance to hit the ball back to either side of the court. Keep your paddle raised and be ready to move your feet to place yourself in a good position to hit the ball back firmly.

When you hit the ball, try to aim for accuracy, and make sure your shot is smooth and precise. Hit the ball back over the net, and either try to aim for the opponent's side closest to the back of the court or the side where they are not as strong. Try not to hit the ball with too much strength because it could cause you to make a mistake. Instead, focus on being accurate and strategic in order to keep your opponents surprised and unsure.

To get better at serving and receiving, you need to practice extensively. Practice your serves on the court and try out different a variety of methods. In the same way, you should practice receiving serves coming from different directions and at different speeds. This will help you get better at returning shots successfully.

Don't forget that serving and receiving aren't just things you do alone; they also require you to work together and correspond with your teammate. Build a good relationship with your teammate and work together to come up with plans that will help you do your best and win in your games.

As you get better at pickleball, serving and receiving will become easy tasks for you. These abilities will be the basic building blocks for your performance in the game and will help you succeed on the pickleball court. Ensure you get plenty of practice, be open to challenges, and have fun while serving and playing pickleball.

Chapter 8: Playing Pickleball With Others

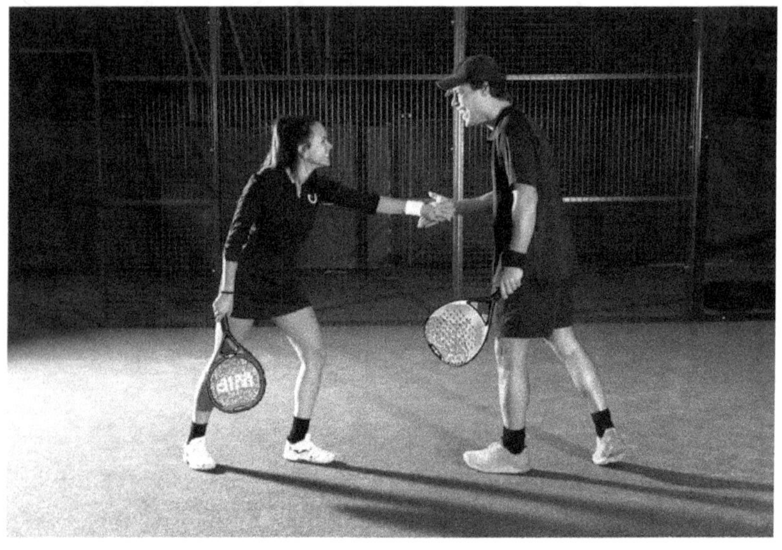

Engaging in pickleball games with fellow players can bring about a deep sense of satisfaction and overall well-being. Not only does it improve your gameplay, but it also aids in meeting new people and forming friendships. When playing pickleball with others, you can expect a different experience, and this chapter aims to provide you with insights into playing together effectively in teams and against opponents.

Playing pickleball alongside others necessitates talking and comprehending each other's perspectives. Having good communication is essential for a smooth game experience and to prevent any misunderstandings, regardless of whether you are playing with a partner or a group.

Utilizing signals, calls, and cues to interact with your teammates can significantly enhance your performance during a game. Effective and straightforward communication ensures mutual understanding and the ability for individuals to anticipate others' actions.

When engaging in group play, it is essential to be conscious of your position on the court. Maintaining the correct position is crucial as it enables you to make better shot choices and prevents unnecessary collisions or obstructions with other players. Gaining an understanding of the various positions and roles within a team can significantly enhance your performance. By collaborating and assuming responsibility for various areas on the court, you can create a formidable and cohesive team.

It is vital to work collectively as a team when participating in pickleball with fellow players. Always bear in mind that your actions have an impact on the overall performance of the group. Hence, never disregard your membership and its significance. Boost the morale of your teammates and offer assistance, commemorate their accomplishments, and offer valuable input as required. By establishing an amicable and co-operative atmosphere within your team, you can elevate your own skills and ensure that the game is a pleasant experience for everyone involved.

While participating in a game, it is crucial to have a clear understanding of your teammates' skills and areas of difficulty. Utilize each other's strengths to your advantage and adapt your playing approach accordingly. Having an understanding of your teammate's playing capabilities, preferences, and strategic thinking fosters improved teamwork. Collaborating and capitalizing on each other's strengths enables your team to enhance its performance and effectively tackle any challenges that arise.

Participating in pickleball with others requires the ability to adapt and modify your approach to each unique situation. Each player possesses a unique playing style and abilities, and embracing the willingness to adapt can enhance enjoyment and performance in the game. Embrace and respect the diversity within your team members while also being willing to adapt your approach by considering the strengths and weaknesses of your competitors. Creating a harmonious and active team dynamic is dependent on your ability to be flexible when playing with others.

Lastly, don't neglect having a wonderful experience. The essence of playing pickleball with other players is not solely centered on competition and winning but on deriving amusement and cultivating camaraderie. Embrace the opportunity to play and enjoy the game, value the moments shared with your teammates, and relish the joy of playing pickleball collectively.

To put it succinctly, participating in pickleball with others provides an entertaining and fulfilling time. In order to have a pleasant and productive time participating in pickleball alongside your teammates, effective communication, proper positioning, teamwork, adaptability, and above all, enjoying yourself are crucial.

The top benefits of playing pickleball and playing the game as a social activity include that it:

- **improves your sleeping patterns:** Doing exercise and engaging in sports can cause certain chemicals in the brain to be released, which can make you feel happier and more relaxed, thereby helping you sleep better. Playing a team sport like pickleball therefore allows you to relieve stress and be part of an activity that helps improve your physical health. If you play the sport outside, the fresh air can also help you sleep better at night.

- **improves your heart:** In order to maintain your strength and good health, it is important to regularly exercise your heart since it functions as a muscle. A strong heart can move blood effectively throughout your body, and your heart will get better at doing its job when you exercise regularly. Improved cardiovascular health contributes to overall physical wellness.

- **serves as a unifying force, like other sports, bringing together people from various communities, backgrounds, religions, and belief systems:** Playing a sport like pickleball can provide an opportunity to meet new people whom you may not usually talk to in ordinary circumstances. Because of this, you are able to encounter and become friends with different people. Playing this sport with a diverse group of individuals can also offer opportunities for new job and business prospects. Additionally, by engaging in this sport with unfamiliar people, you may uncover new employment and entrepreneurial possibilities. Exploring pickleball with a variety of individuals could therefore lead to fresh opportunities that could prove profitable.

- **improve your lung function:** By participating in regular physical activity, the body receives increased oxygen intake and eliminates harmful gases like carbon monoxide and other waste. By enhancing your ability to breathe, participating in physical activity optimizes the performance of your lungs.

- **increase your confidence:** By dedicating ample time to practice and establishing goals for each season, it is possible to boost confidence and enhance your pickleball skills. It becomes evident in tournaments and matches how you and your team showcase your skills. Over time, gaining confidence in yourself can be accomplished through the attainment of small goals. By participating in objective-setting, you will experience an increased sense of competence in tackling new tasks and projects within your professional environment.

- **reduces your stress levels:** When you exercise, your brain gets a break from the worries and pressures of everyday life. Exercising helps your body to decrease stress hormones and increases the release of happy chemicals, called endorphins. These "feel-good" chemicals can make you feel more energized and focused on anything you have to do in life. This is one reason why pickleball is a great choice for you.

- **improves your mental health:** Engaging in sports and maintaining an active lifestyle can be beneficial for enhancing your mental well-being as well. This means that doing this can make you feel happier, more satisfied, and less stressed. It can also help you deal with negative feelings and prevent you from becoming depressed.

- **helps you develop stronger relationships:** Engaging in this sport enables you to develop more profound bonds with individuals you may already be familiar with yet have never encountered in person. Frequent engagement in sports provides valuable insights into an individual's character traits, strengths, and weaknesses. Therefore, engaging in a sporting activity like pickleball with your coworkers also offers a valuable opportunity to foster stronger workplace bonds and connections (*10 Great Benefits of Playing Sport,* 2018).

Grab your paddle, step onto the court, and relish the thrill of playing pickleball alongside fellow enthusiasts.

Chapter 9: Advanced Techniques and Tips

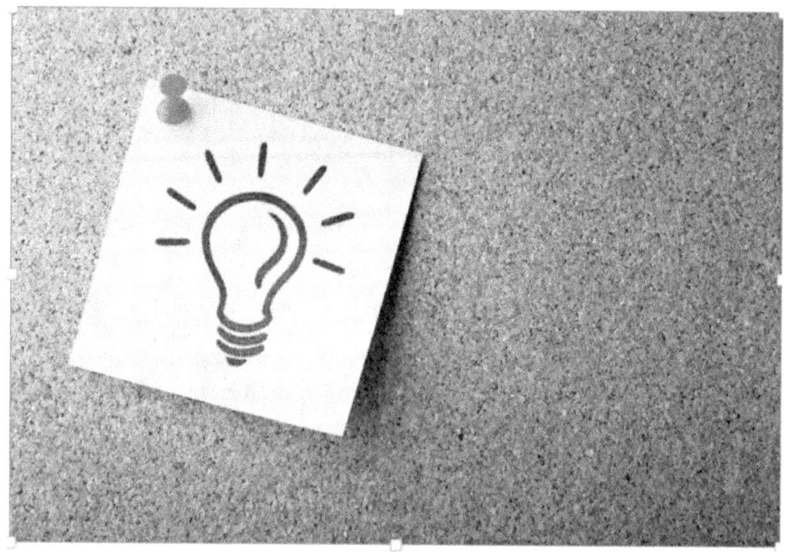

After gaining a solid grasp of pickleball's fundamental rules and getting sufficient practice, it is possible to delve into more advanced techniques. I will explore some of these and provide you with valuable advice to enhance your skills in the game. The following techniques are designed to improve your abilities and enable you to excel in this fun, high-energy game.

Tips and Techniques

Pickleball requires strategy as it entails not only physical strength but also strategic thinking and planning. My main purpose is to provide you with beneficial tactics that can enhance your likelihood of succeeding in the sport. These tips will provide you with an advantage on the court, regardless of whether you're participating in a doubles or singles match. So, let's dive right in!

Master the Third Shot Drop

The third shot drop is a very important move in pickleball, especially when playing with a partner in doubles. This move requires hitting the ball gently and just above the net so that it lands in the opponent's kitchen (non-volley zone). The goal is to hit the ball in a way that makes it hard for your opponents to return the shot, making them hit the ball upward. This gives you a chance to take control of the point. Keep practicing this shot until you do it perfectly, and as a result, you will see your opponents having a hard time returning it.

Develop a Stronger Serve

A good serve in pickleball can help you win. Practice different ways to serve the ball, like hitting it hard, hitting it high, or hitting it with a spin. Always hit the ball hard and at a low trajectory toward the player's weaker hand and within the boundaries of the court.

The game of pickleball is special because players serve the ball by swinging their arms underhand. In simpler words, it's very important to serve accurately in this sport because you only get one chance to get the ball in the right place, unlike in tennis. The serve is the one shot in a pickleball game that you have control over, except for possibly the wind.

So, the serve is a shot in pickleball that you can improve by practicing a lot and becoming very accurate at. When you serve in pickleball, it's not just about getting the ball in the right place. It's crucial to create a situation where your opponents find it difficult to execute a well-aimed return shot. To make it difficult for your opponents to return your serve, try these two suggestions:

Aim for the Weaker Side

In pickleball, aim for your opponent's weaker side, usually their backhand. Most players are better at hitting with their dominant hand than their weaker hand. When serving, hit the ball far into the service box. This will force your opponents to stand farther back and make it harder for them to return the ball. Ideally, this will give you and your partner an advantage for the third shot. However, even though it is generally recommended to hit a deep serve, make sure not to hit the ball out of bounds because you did not leave enough room for mistakes.

Try changing how fast you move, the direction you aim, and where you place shots so that your opponents don't know what to expect. A powerful serve can make your opponent feel stressed right from the beginning and mess up their timing.

Play a Weaker Third Shot

Make your way back to your side of the court and utilize your hand to direct the ball toward your opponent with a weaker third shot. Just like when you serve, when you return the serve in pickleball, you should hit the ball deep into your opponent's side of the court. This means hitting it close to the baseline but still inside the court. This is particularly true if you are playing against a team that likes to hit powerful shots called "bangers."

Hitting the pickleball deep into the court will make it more challenging for the opposing team to return with a powerful shot. This will give you and your partner more time to respond to the play. However, just like the serve, it is usually better to hit a deep return. Make sure you don't hit the return out of bounds because you gave yourself too little room for mistakes. Try to hit your returns in the middle of the court so that you have more room to make up for errors.

You not returning the ball properly gives your opponents an advantage. When you hit the ball back, aim for your opponent's weaker side (usually their backhand) and also target the player on the other team who is not skilled at their third shot. You can do this because, unlike when you serve, you can hit the return of the serve anywhere on your opponent's side of the pickleball court. This means you can focus on one particular player.

In short

- hit your return of serve deep in the court;

- utilize the weaker third shot to hit a member of the opposing doubles team; and

- target the player's weakest side, which is generally their backhand side.

If you have mastered the deep return of serve, then also consider the following, more advanced pickleball strategy tips for the return of serve.

In pickleball, the non-volley-zone line, often referred to as the kitchen line, is where most points are scored. Therefore, it is essential to reach the non-volley-zone line as fast as you can. As the team that is receiving the serve, you need to quickly get to this line after hitting the ball back.

If you're having trouble reaching the non-volley-zone line, try hitting the ball back over the net with a high and arching shot, known as a lob return of serve. This will give you extra time to reach the non-volley zone. Be careful with this plan in two particular situations: When it's windy, the wind can make your shot go out of bounds; and when playing against strong hitters, a high bounce from a lob return may make it easier for them to hit a powerful shot.

Think about adding some spin to how you hit the ball when it's served to you. This will make it harder for your opponents to make a shot. For example, imagine hitting your return of serve with backspin. When you hit the ball back after your opponent's serve, try to hit it with a curved motion so that it spins sideways. This will

- make it harder for your opponents to hit the ball because of the way it spins. Because of the slight reduction in speed caused by the backspin, it is important for both you and your partner to give yourselves additional time in order to reach the non-volley-zone line; and

- make sure to hit the ball close to the ground when it touches the court. Hitting it with topspin will usually make it bounce higher.

If you're playing with someone who always charges to the net and takes the fifth shot in front of their partner, give them the ball to prevent them from crashing the net. Returning the pickleball to its taker will necessitate their second hit, effectively keeping them outside the playing area.

Perfect Your Footwork

This tip may seem easy, but it's actually harder than you think. Many pickleball players forget to adjust their foot position regularly. To do this, you need to move your feet and bend your knees. Your feet play a crucial role in your shots, so it's important to move your feet and position yourself to hit the ball in front of you.

It is important to bend your knees and get close to the ground to effectively hit the low balls in pickleball. This is because keeping the ball down on the court is a key goal. Additionally, when you do this properly, you engage the most powerful muscles in your body, which are your leg muscles.

Good footwork is very important in pickleball because it helps you be in the correct spot to hit the ball effectively. Having good footwork means being able to move your feet quickly and effectively. This will help you to reach difficult shots and stay balanced during intense rallies.

Practice being quick, flexible, and steady to improve your moves during competitive matches. To get better at moving quickly from side to side and reacting fast to your opponents' shots, practice doing quick sideways movements, small jumps called split steps, and quick side-to-side steps called shuffle steps.

Make an effort to tell yourself to move your feet and bend your knees. You might be amazed at how much better you can act and react.

Be Pickleball-Ready

Being picklebally-ready consists of the following:

- standing with your feet a comfortable distance apart, about the width of your shoulders;

- bending your knees and squeezing your body while keeping your weight in the front part of your feet; and

- holding the paddle so that it is pointing toward the front or is at a position that is similar to 10 or 11 o'clock on a clock. If you are left-handed, hold the paddle at a position similar to 1 or 2 o'clock.

Being ready for pickleball is crucial due to the fast-paced nature of the game, especially when approaching the net. To have a better chance of responding quickly to a fast-moving ball, hold your paddle in front of your body. This will help you react with more speed because you don't have to lift your paddle to hit the ball since it's already in position. Stay prepared for the return of the ball, regardless of whether you successfully execute a good shot. Don't get too relaxed, and always expect it to come back to you.

Choose Your Shot and Stick With It

Making decisions on the pickleball court is incredibly important. Having a good understanding of where to aim the ball, adopting a strategic approach that maximizes the likelihood of success, and determining the most advantageous position on are all crucial factors in determining the outcome of a game.

With that being said, it is important to make rapid decisions and stick to the choices you make. Pickleball players sometimes mess up by second-guessing or changing their shot choices. You have a very short amount of time to come to a decision and take a shot. If you decide to change your mind, you are likely to make a mistake because you won't have enough time to make the change properly.

Use Your Strengths and Exploit Your Opponent's Weaknesses

The most important part of any pickleball strategy is to focus on what you are good at and what your opponent is not good at. For example, if you are good at hitting the ball hard and with power, and your opponents are good at playing softly and making short shots, then you should try to hit the ball harder and faster more often. Steer clear of the dinking rallies. Try to lob your opponents if you have a terrific lob and they have a bad overhead or limited movement. Hit to your opponents' backhands if they have strong forehand but poor backhand drives. Utilize your pickleball-court strengths by being aware of them. Discover the flaws of your rivals and take advantage of them!

Keep the Pickleball Low

One of the most challenging things to do in the sport of pickleball is to hit the ball low but still over the net. A low pickleball stops your opponents from making strong shots. For example, if you hit the ball back softly when your opponent serves, they will probably hit the ball softly, too, instead of hitting it hard. Additionally, if you hit the ball low over the non-volley-zone line, it's called a dink instead of a quick volley.

If you hit the pickleball low, it will make your opponents hit it upward. This will give you a chance to hit a powerful shot and score points. The aim for you and your partner in doubles pickleball is to hit the ball close to the ground. To achieve this, think about the angle of your paddle and how hard you hit the pickleball depending on its height.

Use the Correct Paddle Angle

If you hold the paddle upward or level, the pickleball will go higher. Holding the paddle upward toward the sky or keeping it parallel to the net will make the pickleball go lower.

Pace Your Shot

When you hit the ball with a paddle that is open, you slow down the speed of the ball. You can hit the ball slowly so that it stays close to the ground and within the court. When you hit the ball with a paddle that is held at a slant, try to make the ball go faster and aim it down toward the court. Make sure you hit the ball close to the ground, wait for your turn, and take advantage when your opponents hit the ball high up.

Communicate With Your Team

Having effective communication with your partner is a critical tactic for succeeding in a doubles match of pickleball. You and your partner need to talk to each other while playing and in between shots. For example, tell each other who should get the balls in the middle, who will run for the high hits, and if a ball is going out of bounds, say "out" or "bounce it."

Also, talk to your partner during breaks. For example, communicate if your plan needs to change or if either of you notice a weakness in your opponents. Lastly, both of you should talk and support each other. When it comes to being selected for play, this is particularly important when the other team is targeting the player who is not as strong. If you are not chosen to play, your role is to motivate and support your partner while also helping them out whenever you can to reduce their stress. Be a good influence for your partner when playing pickleball. Most people tend to react more favourably to positive things rather than negative things (Townsend, 2021).

Improve Your Dinking Skills

Pickleball requires dinking, which, when done well, has the power to completely alter the course of the game. During dink rallies, practice keeping the ball low and close to the net. To throw off your opponents, try using various dink locations, speeds, and angles. You can manage the tempo of the game and set up winning shots by perfecting the art of this move.

Utilize the Power of the Lob

The lob is a crucial shot that you should use to take back the point or create more options for attack plays. To force your opponents to withdraw to the baseline, practice throwing accurate, high lobs. You'll have the opportunity to advance and seize possession of the net as a result of the court opening up.

Develop a Shot-Placement Strategy

In pickleball, shot placement becomes more crucial as you develop your skill. Concentrate on aiming your shots at particular parts of the court rather than simply sending the ball over the net. Target the corners, weaker side, or sidelines of the opposition to take advantage of their shortcomings. You can manage the pace of the game and keep your opponents on their toes by learning how to place your shots more strategically.

Maintain Mental Focus

At an advanced level, pickleball involves both physical prowess and mental fortitude. Develop the ability to maintain calm and concentration throughout difficult matches. Learn to accept difficulties, maintain optimism, and adjust to various game scenarios. You can make smarter decisions, withstand pressure, and keep your competitive edge by strengthening your mental fortitude.

Remember that it will take time and practice to master these sophisticated strategies and suggestions. To hone your abilities, incorporate them into your training sessions, compete against tough opponents, and attend competitions. You can dominate pickleball matches by outwitting and excelling against your rivals if you put in the effort and persevere.

Now, after learning and implementing all this, you're off to a good start with pickleball!

Conclusion

In the big picture, pickleball is not just a sport but a lifestyle. Within this book, I have delved into the fundamentals, strategies, and methods of this extraordinary and captivating sport. Take some time to learn about the past, the instructions, and the things you need to play. I also made sure to talk about the good things that happen to your body and mind when you play this awesome sport. And now, as we reach the conclusion, I think it's a good opportunity to reflect on some important things.

- Pickleball is a fun sport that anyone, no matter their age or skill, can enjoy. Do not allow your how old you are to hinder your participation.

- Pickleball can be enjoyed by anyone, no matter your fitness level. It doesn't matter if you're a professional athlete or someone who has never worked out before and wants to try a new sport. There is a place for everyone to play. Do not question yourself or think you are not capable enough.

- This game is beautiful because it is easy to play. The rules are simple to comprehend, minimal equipment is required, and the learning process is short. You can immediately dive into this game and experience a positive sense of self.

- I want everyone to remember to be strategic. Despite its initial appearance of simplicity, the game contains additional complexities and proves to be more challenging than expected. In order to achieve victory, understanding your positioning on the court, selecting the appropriate shots, and collaborating effectively with your team are all crucial.

- Through acquiring knowledge about the game and considering diverse scenarios, you have the ability to develop a unique approach and tactics for playing the sport. It is very important to stay concentrated, make quick choices, and adjust to new situations in this fast game.

Building a strong and positive mindset and keeping it during a game can greatly impact the outcome. You can do really well in pickleball when you condition your mind and body.

Pickleball is a sport that brings people together and creates strong relationships, which is something we all need. Whether you're playing in a local league, joining tournaments, or just having friendly matches, this sport unites people.

The common love for pickleball helps people make connections and friendships that go beyond just playing the game. It is a fun activity that you can enjoy with your family, friends, co-workers, or even strangers, and it can create special memories and moments that will stay with you.

One important thing I want you to remember is how crucial it is to become really good at the basics. Just like any other sport, pickleball requires you to have a good set of skills. By practicing holding the equipment correctly, moving your feet properly, and using the right skills appropriately, you can improve your game significantly. To become really great at this sport, you have to practice often and consistently and be committed to getting better.

Pickleball is a game that has something for everyone. I hope you now understand and enjoy this amazing sport more. Regardless of if you are new or experienced in playing pickleball, I urge you to keep discovering and taking advantage of the many opportunities it offers. Get ready with your paddle, go onto the court, and let the game of pickleball make your life better.

References

Introduction to pickleball. (2023). Progress Pickleball. http://www.progresspickleball.com/introduction-to-pickleball.html

Macpherson, R. (2023, April 21). *Beginners guide to pickleball.* Very Well Fit. https://www.verywellfit.com/beginners-guide-to-pickleball-7479881

Nelson, S. (2021, June 28). *An introduction to pickleball.* Restless. https://restless.co.uk/health/healthy-body/an-introduction-to-pickleball/

The strokes and shots of pickleball. (2021, October 26). Badminton Warehouse. https://www.badmintonwarehouse.com/blogs/news/the-strokes-and-shots-of-pickleball

Townsend, S. (2021, February). *Pickleball strategy: 13 tips & techniques to win big.* The Pickler. https://thepickler.com/blogs/pickleball-blog/pickleball-strategy

10 great benefits of playing sport. (2018, March 29). Electric Iceland. https://www.electricireland.com/news/article/10-great-benefits-of-playing-sport

Image References

Absolut Vision. (2017, December 3). *Things to do* [Online image]. Unsplash. https://unsplash.com/photos/82TpEldo_e4

Azeka, J. (2018, April 19). *Pickleball paddles come in some wild colors!* [Online image]. Unsplash. https://unsplash.com/photos/bg43g7xTu2M

Dunn, B. (2020, December 30). *Active wear* [Online image]. Unsplash. https://unsplash.com/photos/EcN3HfcWPxc

Geralt. (2016, October 20). *Rules board* [Online image). Pixabay. https://pixabay.com/illustrations/rules-board-circles-writing-custom-1752415/

Hodskins, P. (2016, June 25). *White shoes* [Online image]. Unsplash. https://unsplash.com/photos/-LoHD3AWwxI

Hoehne, J. (2021, February 16). *The word finish in green turf* [Online image]. Unsplash. https://unsplash.com/photos/Nsaqv7v2V7Q

Klapin, V. (2017, July 20). *Hello!* [Online image]. Unsplash. https://unsplash.com/photos/SymZoeE8quA

Morelli, V. (2022, March 7). *Woman and man rejoice during a paddle match* [Online image]. Unsplash. https://unsplash.com/photos/ZO4pHKtpn4c

Saks, A. (2023, June 14). *Pickleball grip.* [Online image]. Unsplash. https://unsplash.com/photos/a-person-holding-a-baton-with-a-yellow-ball-on-it-CxT3kl4MxAQ

Sidespin. (2022, December 28). *Sidespin paddle* [Online image]. Unsplash. https://unsplash.com/photos/2kvauDh-iuQ

Sigmund. (2020, January 18). *Pixelated game over screen on an oversized PAC-MAN arcade machine* [Online image]. Unsplash. https://unsplash.com/photos/By-tZImtoMs

Tuttle, M. (2023, June 20). *Pickleball paddle, ball, court & net* [Online image]. Pexels. https://www.pexels.com/photo/pickleball-paddle-ball-court-net-17299530/

Views, V. (2021, April 16). *Pickleball* [Online image]. Unsplash. https://unsplash.com/photos/UfnsQzOGLu8

Whitecotton, L. (2022, October 15). *Pickleball game* [Online image]. Unsplash. https://unsplash.com/photos/UHZ_w1bOIvY